Copyright 2021

All right reserved. No part of this book should be reproduced without express permission of the author.

Reproduction of all or any part of this book is punishable under relevant law.

Table of Contents

PREVIEW

Many people consume more calories than they need to maintain their weight each day. When you consistently eat more calories than your body needs, the extra calories are stored as fat.

So how do you get rid of extra fat and lose weight? You create a calorie deficit. This energy deficit happens when you eat less during the day. If your body doesn't get the calories it needs to perform all of its necessary functions, you create a calorie deficit.

When you create a calorie deficit, your body gets energy or fuel from stored fat. This is the extra fat that you carry on your hips or thighs, in your belly, and throughout your body.

Stored fat is stored energy. Your body can use it to keep moving instead of using energy from food. When your body burns fat for energy, you lose weight.

CALORIE DEFICIT DIET RECIPES

BREAKFAST

1. Smoked Salmon Eggs Benedict

Prep Time: 35 Minutes

Cook Time: 5 Minutes

Total Time: 40 Minutes

Yield: 2 Servings

Ingredients

- 4 large eggs
- 2 English muffins, cut in half (Gluten-free, if needed. See notes for Whole30 + paleo)
- 4 tablespoons cream cheese (omit for Whole30 + paleo)
- 3 ounces smoked salmon (salmon lox)
- 2 teaspoons capers
- Thinly sliced red onion
- A pinch of black pepper

Lemony Hollandaise Sauce

- 2 large egg yolks
- 2 tablespoons water
- 2 tablespoons butter (use ghee for Whole30 + paleo)
- 2 teaspoons fresh lemon juice
- A pinch of salt

Instructions

1. Begin by preparing the Hollandaise sauce. Add the egg yolks and water to a small frying pan. Holding the pan 2 inches above an element on medium-high, whisk the eggs until they are frothy and warm. Add the butter to the pan (do not place the pan on the element!) and whisk until the hollandaise is thick. Whisk in the lemon juice and a pinch of salt and set the pan aside.

2. Place a medium-sized pot of water on the stove on high heat.

3. Lightly toast the English muffins either in a toaster or by frying them in a little butter on their cut sides. Place them on the plates you will use to serve them

then spread the cream cheese on top. Divide the smoked salmon between them.

4. When the water comes to a boil, reduce the heat so that it gently simmers. Crack the eggs in one at a time and let them cook for 4 minutes. Remove them from the pot using a slotted spoon and place one egg on top of each English muffin.

5. Pour the hollandaise sauce over the eggs and top with a few slices of red onion, some capers, and a little black pepper.

6. If you're serving this with arugula, toss a few handfuls of baby arugula with a drizzle of olive oil and place the salad beside the eggs benedict.

2. Chai Baked Oatmeal

Prep Time: 10 minutes

Cook Time: 30 minutes

Total Time: 40 minutes

Yield: 6

Ingredients

- 2 cups rolled oats
- 1 can coconut milk (light) (about 1 and ¾ cups)
- 1/4 cup pure maple syrup, plus more for serving
- 1 teaspoon baking powder
- 1/2 teaspoon sea salt
- 1 Tablespoon ground flaxseed
- ½ cup applesauce
- 1 Tablespoon coconut oil
- 1 teaspoon cinnamon
- 1/2 teaspoon cardamom
- 1/2 teaspoon ground ginger
- 1/2 teaspoon allspice
- ⅛ teaspoon cloves
- 1 teaspoon vanilla extract

- 2 Tablespoons shredded coconut
- 2 Tablespoons pecans

Instructions

1. Preheat the oven to 375°F.

2. Spray an 8×8 square baking dish with cooking spray.

3. In a large bowl, mix together the oats, coconut milk, maple syrup, baking powder, sea salt, flaxseed, applesauce, coconut oil, cinnamon, cardamom, ginger, allspice, cloves and vanilla.

4. Carefully pour oatmeal mixture into the prepared baking dish.

5. Scatter pecans and coconut on top.

6. Bake for 25-30 minutes, or until the oatmeal bake has set. Remove from the oven and let cool for a few minutes. Portion and serve with a drizzle of almond milk or maple syrup.

7. For storage: store in the refrigerator in an airtight container for up to 4 days.

8. To reheat: To reheat the whole baked oatmeal, cover with foil and reheat in a 350°F oven for about 20 minutes. For individual portions, set oven (or toaster oven) to 350°F and bake for 5-10 minutes or reheat in the microwave for 1 minute.

3. Hemp Granola

Prep Time: 10 minutes

Cook Time: 65 minutes

Total Time: 1 hour 15 minutes

Yield: 20

Ingredients

- 3/4 cup raw almonds
- 1/2 cup raw pumpkin seeds (pepitas)
- 1/2 cup raw pecans
- 1 cup raw walnuts
- 1 cup unsweetened coconut (desiccated, shredded or flakes)
- 1 cup Manitoba Harvest Hemp Hearts
- 2 Tablespoons chia seeds
- 1/3 cup melted coconut oil
- 1 teaspoon vanilla
- 1 teaspoon cinnamon
- 1/4 cup maple syrup
- pinch of sea salt
- 1/2 cup pitted and chopped Medjool dates

Instructions

1. Preheat oven to 250°F. Place almonds, pumpkin seeds, pecans and walnuts into a food processor and pulse a few times to chop the nuts and seeds into smaller pieces. Don't process too much because you still want some chunky pieces.

2. Transfer the nut mixture into a large bowl, add all remaining ingredients except the dates and stir well. Spread an even layer of the mixture onto a large parchment-lined baking sheet. You may need two sheets if you're baking sheets aren't oversized like mine.

3. Bake for 35 minutes. Remove from oven, add dates and give the mix a good stir. Bake for 25-30 minutes more or until granola is golden brown in color. Remove from oven, let cool and enjoy. It will get crunchier as it cools. I recommend storing any leftovers in a Mason/Weck jar in the fridge. It will stay extra crunchy this way.

4. Easy Shakshuka

Prep Time: 5 minutes

Cook Time: 25 minutes

Total: 30 minutes

Servings: 4

- Ingredients
- 1 Tbsp olive oil 15 mL
- 1 cup diced white onion about 1 medium onion
- 2 cloves garlic minced
- 1 red bell pepper diced
- 2 14.5-oz cans diced tomatoes can sub crushed or whole canned tomatoes
- 1 tsp cumin
- 1tsp smoked paprika
- ¼ tsp each salt and pepper
- 4 to 5 large eggs
- Toppings: feta, parsley (or cilantro), crushed pepper, pita or crusty bread

Instructions

1. Veggies: Preheat oven to 375°F (190°C). Heat oil in an oven-safe skillet over medium heat, then add onion, garlic, and bell pepper. Cook until softened, about 5 minutes.

2. Tomato: Add canned tomatoes, gently mashing them with a fork if needed to form a chunky sauce. Allow tomatoes to simmer, uncovered, until a thick sauce develops, 10 to 15 minutes. Stir in spices, salt, and pepper. Taste and adjust seasonings as needed.

3. Eggs: Using the back of a spoon, form a few holes in the tomato mixture. Crack an egg into each hole (use as many eggs as you want).

4. Bake: Transfer skillet to a preheated oven and cook, uncovered, for 8 to 12 minutes, or until egg whites are mostly cooked. They should be white and still a little jiggly (they'll continue to cook some after removing from the oven). Serve immediately, topped with crumbled feta, herbs, and bread for dipping.

5. Vegan Breakfast Tacos

Prep Time: 10 minutes

Cook Time: 20 minutes

Total Time: 30 minutes

Servings: 6

Ingredients

"Bacon" Chickpeas

- 1 15-oz can chickpeas, drained 425 g
- 1 Tbsp olive oil 15 mL
- 1 Tbsp tamari 15 mL, ca sub soy sauce
- 2 tsp sriracha 10 mL
- 1 tsp maple syrup 5 mL
- 1/2 tsp smoked paprika
- 1/4 tsp each salt and pepper

Roasted Tomatoes:

- 1 cup cherry tomatoes halved, 150 g
- 1 Tbsp olive oil 15 mL
- 1 clove garlic minced

Scrambled Tofu:

- 1 12.3 oz package firm silken tofu 350 g
- 1/4 cup nutritional yeast 20 g
- 2 Tbsp plain hummus 30 g
- 1/4 tsp turmeric
- Pinch salt and pepper

Serving:

- 6 medium flour or corn tortillas
- Garnish with avocado, parsley, lime juice, dairy-free yogurt, sliced radishes

Instructions

1. Roast: Preheat oven to 400 degrees F (204 C). Pat dry chickpeas with paper towels then mix with the rest of the "Bacon" Chickpea ingredients. Spread onto half of a parchment paper-lined baking sheet. Toss together Roasted Tomato ingredients and spread onto the other half. Bake for 20 minutes, or until chickpeas are crispy and tomatoes have burst.

2. Scrambled Tofu: Meanwhile, add all Tofu ingredients to a large greased or non-stick skillet and roughly break up tofu with a spatula. Set over medium heat and cook until tofu begins to brown slightly, stirring often,

3. Assemble: Spoon scrambled tofu, chickpeas, and tomatoes evenly onto tortillas. Garnish with your favorites

6. Delicious Crispy Hash Browns

Prep Time: 15 minutes

Cook Time: 15 minutes

Total Time: 30 minutes

Yield: 4 servings

Ingredients

- 1 pound Russet potatoes (2 small-to-medium), peeled if desired
- ½ teaspoon salt
- ¼ teaspoon garlic powder
- ¼ teaspoon onion powder
- ¼ cup extra-virgin olive oil

Instructions

1. Scrub the potatoes clean and grate them on a large-holed cheese grater (I left the skin on, but you can peel it first if you'd like). In a fine-mesh sieve, rinse the grated potato well until the water runs clear.

2. Drain the potatoes, and then place them potato on a
    clean tea towel or several paper towels. Twist the
    towel to remove as much moisture from the potatoes
    as possible (you might need to do this in two batches).

3. Transfer the grated potato to a bowl and toss it with
    the salt, garlic powder and onion powder.

4. In a large skillet (preferably cast iron, but non-stick
    works, too), warm the olive oil over medium heat until
    shimmering and a piece of grated potato sizzles on
    contact. Spread the potatoes over the skillet in an even
    layer and press them down with a spatula. Let them
    cook, undisturbed, for 2 minutes.

5. Stir again, press them down again, and cook for
    another 2 minutes. Repeat in 2-minute intervals,
    flipping in sections once they're crispy enough to do
    so, until the potatoes are golden brown and crispy,
    about 4 to 8 more minutes. Meanwhile, line a plate
    with a couple of layers of paper towels to absorb
    excess oil, and set it near the stove.

6. Transfer the hash browns to the lined plate and let them drain for a minute. (If you're making multiply batches of hash browns, repeat these steps as necessary—keep in mind that your skillet will be really hot so your next batch may cook faster.)

7. Season to taste with additional salt, if necessary, and serve hot.

7. Homemade Bircher Muesli

Prep Time: 10 minutes

Cook Time: 0 minutes

Total Time: 10 minutes

Yield: 1 serving

Ingredients

- ⅓ cup old-fashioned oats
- 1 tablespoon raisins or dried cranberries or cherries
- ¼ teaspoon ground cinnamon
- 1 tablespoon almond butter or peanut butter
- 2 tablespoons homemade applesauce or store-bought applesauce
- ⅓ cup milk of choice (I used almond milk), plus extra for serving (optional)
- 1 medium Granny Smith or Honeycrisp apple, preferably organic
- Chopped pecans, walnuts or almonds
- Drizzle of honey or maple syrup, if desired

Instructions

1. In a jar or bowl (a 14-ounce working jar or 1-pint mason jar is perfect), combine the oats, raisins, cinnamon, nut butter and applesauce. Stir to combine. Then add the milk and stir to combine.

2. Grate half of the apple, then stir the grated apple into the oatmeal (if you're making multiple jars, just use 1 grated apple for 2 jars, and so on).

3. Place the lid on the jar and refrigerate for at least 30 minutes, or up to 5 days. When you're ready to serve, chop the remaining ½ apple into matchsticks. Top the oatmeal with the fresh apple, a splash of milk and/or a drizzle of honey (both optional). Enjoy chilled.

8. Tropical Acai Bowl

Prep Time: 10 minutes

Cook Time: 0 minutes

Total Time: 10 minutes

Yield: 2 smoothie bowls

Ingredients

- 1 ½ cups frozen mango chunks
- 1 cup frozen pineapple chunks
- 1 cup frozen banana chunks (freeze ripe bananas in ½"-thick slices)
- Two packets (3.5 ounces or 100 grams each) frozen unsweetened açai berry purée
- 1 cup ice cold water, more if necessary
- 1 to 2 tablespoons lime juice, to taste
- Recommended garnishes: coconut granola, shredded unsweetened coconut, chopped nuts, chia seeds, sliced fresh banana or kiwi or other tropical fruits

Instructions

1. In a blender, combine the frozen mango, pineapple and banana. Run the açaí packets under warm water for about 10 seconds to let them thaw a bit, then cut them open and pour the açaí pulp into the blender.

2. Pour in the cold water, securely fasten the lid, and start blending on the lowest speed until you can gain traction, increasing to high speed as it becomes available. If necessary, pause the blender to scrape down the sides, and add ¼ cup to ½ cup more water if it just won't blend.

3. Add 1 to 2 tablespoons lime juice, to taste, and blend briefly to combine. Pour the smoothie into bowls and top with garnishes of your choice. Serve immediately, or cover and refrigerate for up to 3 days.

9. Cheesy Potato Fritters with Zucchini

Prep Time:15 minutes

Cook Time:20 minutes

Total Time:35 minutes

Servings: 14

Ingredients

- 3 cups shredded zucchini about 13 ounces or 2 medium
- 2 cups shredded Yukon gold potatoes about 12 ounces or 2 small/medium, scrubbed and peeled
- 1/2 medium yellow onion shredded
- 3 large eggs lightly beaten
- 1/2 cup seasoned whole wheat breadcrumbs
- 1/3 cup white whole wheat flour or substitute all-purpose flour
- 1 teaspoon garlic powder
- 1 teaspoon kosher salt plus additional to season
- 1/2 teaspoon ground black pepper
- 1 teaspoon baking soda
- 1/2 cup freshly grated sharp cheddar cheese

- 1-2 tablespoons olive oil for frying
- Plain nonfat Greek Yogurt for serving
- Chopped fresh chives for serving

Instructions

1. If you'd like to keep the fritters warm between batches, preheat your oven to 200 degrees F. Spread the shredded zucchini, potatoes, and onion onto a clean kitchen towel and press out as much moisture as possible, changing the towel once or twice as needed.

2. Place the shredded vegetables in a large bowl, then add the eggs, breadcrumbs, flour, garlic powder, salt, pepper, and baking soda. Mix until completely combined, using your fingers if needed to make sure all of the ingredients are evenly distributed. Fold in the shredded cheese.

3. In a large nonstick skillet, heat 1 tablespoon of the olive oil over medium heat. Scoop a scant 1/4-cup portion of the fritter batter onto the frying pan and flatten into an even layer, using either the back of the measuring spoon or the bottom of a drinking glass. Cook for 3 to 4 minutes until golden on the first side,

then flip and continue cooking until the second side is golden as well. Depending upon your skillet, you may need to adjust the heat as you go to ensure the pancakes cook all the way through but still get crisp on the outside. Repeat with the remaining pancakes, keeping batches warm in the oven as desired. If excess liquid collects in the bottom of the bowl, discard it. Serve warm, topped with Greek yogurt and fresh chives.

10. Bagel Egg in a Hole with Smashed Avocado

Prep Time: 5 minutes

Cook Time: 10 mintes

Total Time: 15 minutes

Servings: 2

Ingredients

- 1 whole grain bagel
- 1 tablespoon unsalted butter, softened
- 2 large eggs
- 1 small ripe Hass avocado
- 1/4 teaspoon kosher salt plus additional to taste
- 1/8 teaspoon black pepper
- 1/4 teaspoon red pepper flakes optional
- Chopped fresh herbs: cilantro parsley, chives,

Instructions

1. Slice bagel in half. If the hole is very small, tear out some of the center to make it larger or use a round cookie cutter, small juice glass, or biscuit cutter to cut

a larger hole. Lightly spread the cut sides of the bagel with butter. In a small bowl, mash the avocado with the salt, black pepper, and red pepper flakes (if using). Taste and add additional seasoning if desired.

2. For each bagel half: Heat a non-stick skillet over medium. Place the bagel in the skillet butter-side down. Let toast a few minutes until golden, then flip and place on a plate, toasted side up. Spread the cut side with mashed avocado. Return the bagel to the skillet, avocado-side up. Crack an egg in the center of the hole (for easier transfer, you can also crack the egg in a small bowl, then gently pour it into the hole), then cover the skillet and let cook until the egg is set, about 3 minutes for a medium-soft yolks (if your skillet does not have a lid, you can also place a sheet pan over the top—the idea is to trap heat to cook the egg more quickly). Transfer to a serving plate, sprinkle with any desired toppings. Enjoy immediately.

LUNCH

11. Caribbean Bowls With Jerk Shrimp

Prep Time: 15 minutes

Cook Time: 25 minutes

Total Time: 40 minutes

Yield: 6

Ingredients

- 1 16 oz package of frozen sweet plantains
- 1 ½ cups jasmine rice
- 1 teaspoon salt (optional)
- 2 lbs of peeled and deveined shrimp
- 3–4 Tablespoons jerk seasoning
- Hot sauce, for serving
- fresh cilantro, for garnish
- cilantro lime dressing or tomatillo dressing, for serving (optional)

Pineapple Salsa:

- 1 15 oz can of black beans, drained and rinsed

- 1 cup chopped pineapple (fresh is best but thawed frozen works too)
- 1 cup chopped cherry tomatoes
- ½ cup diced red onion
- ¼ cup chopped cilantro + more for topping
- 1–2 Tablespoon diced jalapeno
- 2 limes, juiced
- ½ teaspoon sea salt
- Pinch of pepper

Instructions

1. Roast plantains: Roast plantains according to package instructions. You can use the oven or the air-fryer for this!

2. Make rice: While plantains are roasting, prepare rice: sort and rinse rice before cooking. Combine 1 ½ cups rice with 3 cups water in a large pot. Add 1 teaspoon salt, if using. Bring to a boil. Reduce heat, cover with lid and simmer for 15 minutes. Remove from heat, fluff with a fork and keep warm until ready to serve.

3. Make pineapple salsa: add pineapple, black beans, tomatoes, onion, cilantro, jalapeño, salt, pepper and lime juice in a bowl. Toss to combine.

4. Cook shrimp: toss shrimp with jerk seasoning. In a large skillet, heat oil over medium-high heat. Add shrimp; cook and stir until shrimp turn pink, 2-3 minutes. Remove from heat.

5. Serve: place rice in each bowl, top with shrimp, a scoop of black bean pineapple mixture, and 3-4 roasted plantains. Garnish with cilantro, hot sauce and dressing, if using.

12. Greek Salad

Prep Time: 15 minutes

Total Time: 15 minutes

Yield: 4

Ingredients

- 1 head of romaine lettuce, chopped
- ½ cup red onion, halved and sliced
- 1 cup grape or cherry tomatoes, halved
- ½ English cucumber, thinly sliced and halved
- ½ cup chopped cubes of fresh feta or crumbled feta
- ¼ cup pitted kalamata olives, halved
- Optional additions: avocado, chopped bell pepper, pepperoncini peppers, chickpeas or grilled chicken

Greek Salad Dressing

- 2 small garlic cloves, minced
- 1 teaspoon dijon mustard
- 1 teaspoon dried oregano
- 2 Tablespoons red wine vinegar
- juice of 1 lemon (about 2–3 Tablespoons)

- ¼ cup olive oil
- ½ teaspoon salt
- ½ teaspoon black pepper

Instructions

1. Make dressing: place all ingredients for the dressing except olive oil. Blend and then slowly add in olive oil while blending on low. You can also do this with an immersion blender. Set aside.

2. Prep lettuce: Rinse, chop and dry romaine lettuce. I like using my salad spinner to dry it. Transfer chopped lettuce to a large salad bowl.

3. Add toppings: Add red onion, tomatoes, cucumber, olives and feta cheese. Add additional topping options, if desired.

4. Add dressing: Drizzle half of the dressing over the salad, toss and taste. Add more dressing, if needed.

13. Chicken Fajita Soup

Prep Time: 20 minutes

Cook Time: 4 hours

Total Time: 4 hours 20 minutes

Yield: 4

Ingredients

- 1 yellow bell pepper, chopped
- 1 orange bell pepper, chopped
- 1 green bell pepper, chopped
- 1 medium yellow onion, chopped
- 1/2 jalapeño pepper, sliced
- 1 cup fresh salsa
- 2 cloves garlic, minced
- juice of 1 lime
- 4 cups low-sodium vegetable or chicken broth
- 1 1/2 pound boneless skinless chicken thighs (chicken breasts work too)
- 1 teaspoon olive oil
- 1 Tablespoon chili powder
- 1 teaspoon cumin

- 1 teaspoon paprika
- 1 teaspoon sea salt
- 1 teaspoon ground pepper
- cauliflower rice or cooked white/brown rice (optional)
- toppings of choice: chopped avocado, jalapeño slices, cilantro, more lime juice, tortilla chips or crackers

Instructions

Slow Cooker:

1. Put all ingredients (besides rice and toppings) into a slow cooker.

2. Cook for 3-4 hours on high or 6 hours on low. The chicken should be cooked through and will just fall apart. Once this happens turn the slow cooker to warm and enjoy whenever you're ready. If adding rice, add it to the slow cooker while set to warm.

3. To serve, top each bowl with avocado, jalapeño slices, cilantro and serve with tortilla chips and a slice of lime.

Instant Pot / Pressure Cooker:

1. Add olive oil to Instant Pot and put on sauté setting. Add onion and garlic and sauté for about 5 minutes, until fragrant.

2. Add remaining ingredients (besides rice and toppings). Place the lid on the pressure cooker, lock lid and make sure the pressure release valve is closed.

3. Press cancel on the pressure cooker and then press the soup/stew button and set time to 30 minutes.

4. Once the timer reaches 0, the cooker will switch to keep warm. Carefully switch the pressure release valve to open to manually release the pressure. (I use tongs for this). Once the steam is released, remove the lid and use a fork to shredded chicken. The chicken should be cooked through and will just fall apart.

5. If adding rice, add it to the Instant Pot while set to warm. Once warm throughout, portion soup into bowls.

6. To serve, top each bowl with avocado, jalapeño slices, cilantro and serve with tortilla chips and a slice of lime.

14. Cauliflower Pizza Crust

Prep Time: 15 minutes

Cook Time: 35 minutes

Total Time: 50 minutes

Yield: 2-4

Ingredients

Crust:

- 2 cups riced cauliflower (about ½ head)
- 1 clove garlic, minced
- 1 cup part-skim shredded mozzarella cheese
- 1 egg, beaten
- 1 teaspoon dried basil
- 1 teaspoon dried oregano
- Olive oil spray or 1 teaspoon olive oil, for greasing

Toppings:

- ⅓ cup pizza sauce
- 1 cup part-skim shredded mozzarella cheese
- Fresh basil

- Crushed red pepper

Instructions

1. Preheat oven: Preheat oven to 400° F.

2. Prep a baking sheet or pizza stone: Line a baking sheet or pizza stone with parchment. Grease the parchment with olive oil spray or rub on regular olive oil.

3. Prep cauliflower: If using whole cauliflower, remove the stems and leaves from the cauliflower and chop the florets into chunks. Add to a food processor or blender and pulse just until the texture is similar to rice. If you don't have a food processor or high powered blender, you can grate the cauliflower with a cheese grater or chop it. Another (much faster option) is to buy riced cauliflower.

4. Cook cauliflower rice: Sauté cauliflower "rice" in a non-stick skillet over medium heat and cook until translucent, approximately 6-8 minutes. (You can use the microwave for this as well. Just place cauliflower

in an uncovered microwave-safe bowl and cook for 8 minutes.)

5. Mix cauliflower dough: In a bowl combine the cooked cauliflower with garlic, mozzarella cheese, egg, basil and oregano. The cheese will melt a bit and this is okay.

6. Spread dough to make the crust: Spread dough out evenly on your parchment lined baking sheet and form into a circle. You'll want it to be about 1/4 to 1/3 of an inch thick. The pizza should be about 9-10 inches in diameter.

7. Bake: Bake for 25-30 minutes or until the crust is golden, crispy on the edges and cooked through the middle.

8. Remove the crust from the oven and set oven to broil.

9. Add toppings: Top with pizza sauce and cheese. You can also add additional toppings, but be careful not to add too many heavy toppings as you don't want to weigh down the crust.

10. Broil: Broil the pizza for 5 minutes, or until the toppings are hot and the cheese is melted. Allow the pizza to cool for 2-3 minutes then cut and serve immediately. Serve with fresh basil and crushed red pepper.

15. Healthy Taco Salad

Prep Time: 25 minutes

Cook Time: 30 minutes

Total Time: 55 minutes

Yield: 3

Ingredients

Turkey Taco Meat:

- 12 mini bell peppers
- olive or avocado oil spray
- 1/2 Tablespoon olive oil
- 1 lb ground turkey
- 2 Tablespoons taco seasoning
- 2 Tablespoons fresh salsa

Salad:

- 1 large head romaine lettuce, washed, rinsed, dried and chopped
- 1/2 cup grape or cherry tomatoes, chopped
- 1/2 cup thawed frozen sweet corn

- 1/4 cup shredded Mexican cheese + more to taste
- 1/2 jalapeño pepper, de-seeded and chopped (optional)
- 1 avocado, chopped into chunks
- 1/4 cup tortilla chips, broken into pieces
- chopped cilantro, for garnish
- hot sauce, to taste (optional)
- fresh salsa, to taste

Creamy Southwest Dressing:

- 4 ounces plain Greek yogurt
- 1 teaspoons lime juice
- 1/8 teaspoon cumin
- 1/4 teaspoon chili powder
- 1/4 teaspoon garlic powder
- 1/4 teaspoon salt
- 1/4 teaspoon pepper
- 1/4 cup fresh salsa
- 2 Tablespoons fresh cilantro

Instructions

1. Roast peppers: Preheat oven to 400°F. Place peppers
    on a baking sheet, spray with olive or avocado oil
    cooking spray, sprinkle on a little salt and pepper and
    place in the oven to roast for 20-30 minutes, or until
    peppers are soft. Let peppers cool, remove stems and
    any large seeds and then dice into small pieces. The
    diced up peppers should measure out to be about 1/3
    cup.

2. Make dressing: Add all ingredients for the dressing
    into a blender and blend until fully combined and
    smooth. You can also use an immersion blender for
    this.

3. Cook turkey: Add oil to a skillet over medium heat.
    Once hot, add turkey. Break meat into small pieces
    using a spatula or meat chopper as it cooks. Cook for
    about 6-8 minutes or until the turkey is no longer
    pink. Add taco seasoning, salsa and roasted peppers
    to the pan and toss to combine. Set aside.

4. Prep salads: While the turkey it cooking start to prep
    your salad ingredients. To build salads, start with a

base of romaine lettuce in each bowl and add the toppings — turkey taco meat, tomatoes, corn, cheese, jalapeño, avocado and chips.

5. Serve: Drizzle a little dressing over each salad and serve with chopped cilantro and extra dressing. Add some fresh salsa and a few drops of hot sauce if using. Another option is to place all the salad ingredients into a large salad bowl and toss with dressing, then portion into two-four bowls for serving.

16. Roasted Vegetable Salad

Prep Time: 20 minutes

Cook Time: 40 minutes

Total Time: 1 hour

Yield: 4

Ingredients

- 2 cups cauliflower florets, bite-size
- 2 cups butternut squash chunks
- 3 cups Brussels sprouts, halved
- 1 15 oz. can cannellini beans (rinsed and drained)
- 1/4 cup fresh pomegranate arils or dried pomegranate seeds
- 3 Tablespoons dried mulberries
- 4 cups thinly sliced Lacinato (dinosaur) kale
- Olive or avocado oil (or spray)

Dressing:

- 3 Tablespoons champagne vinegar*
- 1 Tablespoon prepared horseradish
- 1 clove garlic, minced

- 2 teaspoons minced scallions
- 1 pinch crushed red pepper flakes
- 1 teaspoon sea salt
- ⅓ cup extra virgin olive oil

Instructions

1. Roast veggies: Heat oven to 400°F. Place cauliflower, butternut squash and brussels sprouts on a large baking sheet, spray with a little avocado oil spray or drizzle with oil, sprinkle with salt and pepper and toss to combine. Roast for 30-40 minutes or until veggies are until well caramelized and softened with a few golden brown spots. Stir once mid-way through the cooking process and watch closely so the veggies don't burn.

2. Prep dressing: While veggies are cooking, make the dressing: Combine all ingredients except the olive oil and whisk to combine. Slowly drizzle in the olive oil while whisking, set aside. Taste and add more olive oil, if needed.

3. Prep salad: Remove vegetables from oven and allow to cool to room temperature, then combine in a large

bowl with the beans, kale and pomegranate seeds. Toss in the dressing to evenly coat everything. You may find that you don't need to use all of the dressing.

4. Serve: Portion into bowls, top with mulberries and serve.

5. Store: Salad will keep marinated for up to 2 days in the fridge.

17. Low Carb Baked Feta Pasta

Cook Time: 40 minutes

Total Time: 40 minutes

Yield: 4

Ingredients

- 16 oz cherry tomatoes
- 8 oz block feta, packed in water
- ⅓ cup olive oil
- ½ teaspoon sea salt
- ¼ teaspoon black pepper
- 1–2 large garlic cloves, minced
- ¼ cup fresh chopped basil, plus more for serving
- 1 teaspoon lemon zest
- ½ teaspoon crushed red pepper, plus more for serving
- 1 medium spaghetti squash (about 4 cups)
- cracked black pepper and fresh parmesan, for serving

Instructions

1. Preheat oven to 400°F.

2. Cook squash: Start cooking your spaghetti squash using my spaghetti squash recipe. The squash cooks at 400°F as well so you can easily bake the squash and feta at the same time. Just put the squash in about 20-30 minutes before you add the feta in because the squash takes a bit longer to cook and you have to pull the strands from it as well.

3. Prep tomatoes and feta: Add cherry tomatoes to a rectangular baking dish and nestle the block of feta in the middle. Drizzle olive oil over the tomatoes and feta. Sprinkle on salt and pepper and use a spoon to toss until all of the tomatoes are coated.

4. Bake: Place in the oven for 30 minutes or until tomatoes are sizzling and feta has softened.

5. Season and mix: Bring dish out of the oven and sprinkle on the fresh chopped basil, minced garlic (roasted garlic would be even better), lemon zest and crushed red pepper, if using. Stir the mixture until everything is well combined.

6. Add squash noodles: Measure out 4 cups of cooked spaghetti squash and add to the baking dish with the baked feta and tomatoes. Use a spoon to toss until all the strands of spaghetti squash are coated.

7. Serve: Portion pasta and serve with extra chopped basil, crushed red pepper, cracked black pepper and fresh parmesan.

18. Instant Pot Garlic Lentil Soup

Prep Time: 15 minutes

Cook Time: 30 minutes

Total Time: 45 minutes

Yield: 10 cups

Ingredients

- 3 Tablespoons olive oil
- 1 sweet yellow onion, chopped
- 2 carrots, chopped
- 2 stalks celery, chopped
- 1 bulb roasted garlic (about 8–10 cloves), chopped
- 1– 16 oz bag dry French green or brown lentils, sorted and rinsed
- 2 (32 oz) containers of low-sodium vegetable broth
- 1 (14.5 oz) can diced tomatoes
- 1 Tablespoon tomato paste
- 1 teaspoon dried oregano
- ½ teaspoon dried thyme
- 1/2 teaspoon paprika
- 1/2 teaspoon cumin

- pinch of nutmeg

- 2 bay leaves

- 1 teaspoon sea salt + more to taste

- 1 teaspoon ground pepper + more to taste

- 2 Tablespoons red wine vinegar

- Optional toppings: sriracha, avocado, fresh parsley

Instructions

1. Instant Pot/Pressure Cooker.

2. Using the sauté function on high, heat oil in the inner pot for about 1 minute, until shimmering. Add the onion, carrots, celery and cook for about 5 minutes, until fragrant and onions are turning translucent. Season with a little salt and pepper while cooking.

3. Stir in the roasted garlic, lentils, broth, diced tomatoes, tomato paste, oregano, thyme, paprika, cumin, nutmeg, bay leaves, salt and pepper. Secure the lid and cook on high pressure for 15 minutes.

4. Once the cooking is complete, let the pressure release naturally for 10 minutes, then quick-release the remaining pressure.

5. Remove bay leaves, stir in vinegar, taste and add additional salt and pepper, if needed.

6. Ladle soup into bowls and serve with toppings of choice. I personally love adding fresh parsley and a splash of sriracha.

Stove-Top

1. Heat oil in a large soup pot over medium-high heat. Add the onion, carrots and celery to the pot, stirring frequently for 8-10 minutes or until onions are soft and translucent. Season with a little salt and pepper while cooking.

2. Add roasted garlic, lentils, broth, diced tomatoes, vinegar, tomato paste, oregano, thyme, paprika, cumin, nutmeg, bay leaves, salt and pepper.

3. Bring to a boil, then reduce heat, cover and simmer, stirring every so often, for at least 1 hour or until the lentils are soft.

4. Remove bay leaves, stir in vinegar, taste and add additional salt and pepper, if needed.

5. Ladle soup into bowls and serve with toppings of choice. I personally love adding fresh parsley and a splash of sriracha.

19. Butternut Squash Quinoa Stuffing

Prep Time: 10 minutes

Cook Time: 15 minutes

Total Time: 25 minutes

Yield: 4 servings

Ingredients

- 1 Tablespoon vegan butter (regular butter works too)
- 1 yellow onion, peeled and chopped
- 3 cloves garlic, minced
- 1/2 cup celery, chopped
- 3 cups peeled and chopped butternut squash
- 8 oz package of baby bella mushrooms, chopped
- 1/3 cup vegetable broth or bone broth
- 1 1/2 cups dry quinoa, rinsed and drained
- 3 cups water
- 1 bay leaf
- 2 Tablespoons chopped fresh sage
- 1 teaspoon dried thyme
- 1 teaspoon dried parsley
- 1/2 teaspoon sea salt

- 1/2 teaspoon ground pepper
- 1/3 cup chopped pecans
- 1/4 cup dried cranberries or cherries
- more sea salt and pepper, to taste

Instructions

1. Cook quinoa: Add quinoa, water and bay leaf into a saucepan. Bring mixture to a boil, reduce to a simmer, cover and cook for 15 minutes or until all the water is absorbed and quinoa is fluffy. Remove bay leaf.

2. Cook veggies: Heat butter in a large skillet. Add onion, garlic and celery and sauté until onion is fragrant and translucent, about 5-7 minutes. Add mushrooms and cook for another 1-2 minutes. Add butternut squash, broth, sage, thyme, parsley, salt and pepper to the pan. Cover and let mixture cook for about 5 minutes, then remove top and simmer for another 10 minutes, allowing most of the broth to evaporate. You'll know it's done when the butternut squash is cooked through and fork tender. Remove from heat.

3. Mix Everything Together: Add cooked quinoa into a large bowl and top with cooked veggie mixture and dried cranberries to the quinoa. Stir to combine, taste and add more salt and pepper, if needed.

4. Bake: Preheat oven to 375°F. Transfer mixture into a 9×13 baking dish, top with chopped pecans and bake for 20 minutes or until pecans are golden brown and toasted. Serve warm.

20. Tuna Stuffed Bell Peppers

Prep Time: 10 minutes

Cook Time: 20 minutes

Total Time: 30 minutes

Yield: 2

Ingredients

- 2 medium bell peppers (orange, yellow or red)
- 1/3 cup red onion, chopped into small pieces
- 2 button mushrooms, chopped into small pieces
    - 5-oz. can water-packed tuna
- 1/2 cup chopped cherry tomatoes
- 1/4 cup chopped kalamata olives
- 1/4 cup no salt added cottage cheese (I use the Friendship brand)
    - Tablespoon fresh lemon juice
- 1 teaspoon extra virgin olive oil
- 1/2 teaspoon dijion mustard
- 1/2 teaspoon dried parsley
- 1/2 teaspoon dried oregano
- crushed red pepper (optional)

- freshly ground black pepper
- sea salt

Instructions

1. Preheat oven to broil. Place whole peppers onto a baking stone or sheet and broil for 5-7 minutes, turning once mid-way through broiling. Watch the peppers carefully so you don't complete char them. Remove from the heat, and place on a plate to cool.

2. Turn oven from broil to 350°F.

3. While waiting for the peppers to cool, make your tuna filling. Spray a skillet with cooking spray and sauté the onions and mushrooms until soft and fragrant, sprinkle with sea salt and black pepper while cooking.

4. Add cooked onion and mushroom into a medium size mixing bowl.

5. Add tuna, tomatoes, olives, cottage cheese, lemon juice, olive oil, mustard, parsley and oregano to the bowl as well. Break apart tuna with a fork and stir all the ingredients together. Season to taste with crushed

red pepper and ground pepper (it should not need any additional salt).

6. Once the broiled peppers are cool enough to handle, carefully cut the peppers in half, remove seeds and membranes (be careful as it may still be hot inside). Lay the 4 pepper halves on the baking stone and fill with the tuna mixture. You should have just enough tuna to fill the 4 pepper halves. If you have extra, you can eat it on the side or save it for later.

7. Place peppers in the oven for 10-15 minutes, until warm all the way through. Remove from oven, serve and enjoy.

DINNER

21. Roasted Tomato Salad

Prep Time: 15 minutes

Cook Time: 45 minutes

Total Time: 1 hour 15 minutes

Yield: 4

Ingredients

- 2 lbs tomatoes cherry tomatoes, halved (about 6 cups chopped tomatoes)
- 1/4 cup olive oil
- Tablespoon maple syrup
- 1/2 teaspoon sea salt
- 3/4 cup diced cucumber
- 1/2 cup feta, cut or crumbled into small chunks*
- 1/4 cup red onion, chopped
- Tablespoons white balsamic vinegar
- Tablespoon fresh basil, finely chopped
- sea salt and pepper, to taste

Instructions

1. Preheat the oven to 350°F and adjust one of your oven racks to the top third of the oven.

2. Cut tomatoes in half and place 1 pound in a bowl, set aside.

3. Gently toss the other pound of tomatoes in a bowl with the olive oil, maple syrup, and salt. Arrange them in a single layer, cut side up, on a rimmed baking sheet.

4. Bake until the tomatoes shrink and start to caramelize around the edges, about 45 minutes. Set tomatoes aside to cool for 30 minutes.

5. Gently toss roasted tomatoes, fresh tomatoes, cucumber, feta cheese, onion, vinegar and basil in large bowl. Sprinkle with sea salt and ground pepper to taste.

22. Spaghetti Squash Pad Thai

Prep Time: 20 minutes

Cook Time: 45 minutes

Total Time: 1 hour 5 minutes

Yield: 4 servings

Ingredients

- large spaghetti squash (approx. 5 cups after roasting)
- Tablespoon + 2 teaspoons olive or avocado oil
  - 1 lb boneless skinless chicken breast
  - Sea salt and ground pepper
  - ½ teaspoon chopped ginger
  - ½ cup chopped yellow onion
  - 1 sliced red bell pepper
  - 1 cup matchstick carrots
  - Green onions, fresh cilantro and lime wedges, for garnish
  - Tablespoons chopped salted almonds (optional)

Chili Almond Sauce:

- ½ cup natural almond butter (no sugar added)

- 2 Tablespoons fresh lime juice
- Tablespoon low sodium tamari or coconut aminos
- inch knob fresh ginger, peeled
- cloves garlic
- teaspoons maple syrup
- 1 teaspoon sambal oelek or crushed red pepper
- ¼ cup water

Instructions

1. Cook spaghetti squash in rings using instructions from my spaghetti squash post.

2. Allow squash rings to cool for about 15 minutes, then peel the skin away and use a fork to separate the strands.

3. While squash is roasting, make the chili almond sauce by adding all ingredients into a blender or food processor. Process until smooth and set aside.

4. Chop raw chicken breasts into 1-inch chunks. Heat a large skillet over medium heat with 1 Tablespoon oil. Add chicken to the skillet and liberally season

with sea salt and pepper. Cook, stirring often until all sides are golden and chicken is cooked through and no longer pink. Transfer to a plate and set aside.

5. Add remaining 2 teaspoons of oil to the same skillet and sauté together ginger, onion, bell pepper and carrots. Cook until the veggies are starting to soften, about 5-6 minutes.

6. Add chicken back to the skillet with the veggies. Then add the chili almond sauce and mix everything together thoroughly.

7. Add spaghetti squash to the skillet and mix again. If your skillet isn't large enough, you can put everything in a large bowl to mix instead.

8. Serve the spaghetti squash pad Thai immediately with green onions, fresh cilantro and lime wedges for garnish. Top with chopped almonds.

23. Red Beans And Rice

Prep Time: 10 minutes

Cook Time: 18 minutes

Total Time: 28 minutes

Yield: 4

Ingredients

- 2 Tablespoons olive oil
- 2 cups chopped yellow onion
- 4 stalks of celery, chopped
- large green bell pepper, chopped
- cup sliced carrots
- 8 garlic cloves, minced
- 1 bay leaf
- teaspoons paprika
- 1 teaspoon dried thyme
- 1 teaspoon dried oregano
- ½ teaspoon onion powder
- ½ teaspoon garlic powder
- 1 ½ teaspoons sea salt
- ½ teaspoon pepper

- ½ teaspoon crushed red pepper
- Shake of cayenne pepper (optional)
- 1 tablespoon red wine vinegar
- cups cooked red kidney beans (drained and rinsed if using canned)
- 1 cup vegetable broth + more if needed
- cooked rice, for serving
- fresh flat-leaf parsley, for garnish

Instructions

1. Heat a large nonstick skillet over medium-high. Add oil. Once hot, add your onion, celery, bell pepper, carrot and garlic. Cook until onion is translucent and mixture is fragrant, about 10 minutes. Add in bay leaf, paprika, thyme, oregano, onion powder, garlic powder, sea salt, pepper and crushed red pepper. Toss to combine and then add red wine vinegar to the pan. Reduce heat.

2. While veggies are cooking, mash 1/2 cup of the red beans with a fork.

3. Add mashed beans, remaining 2 1/2 cups whole beans and vegetable broth to the pan. Bring mixture to a simmer and cook for about 8 minutes or until vegetables are tender, stirring occasionally. If mixture seems too thick, add a splash of more vegetable broth to thin it out a bit. Taste and season with additional salt and pepper, if needed.

4. Add rice to bowls and top each with bean mixture. Sprinkle with fresh parsley and serve.

24. Chicken Wild Rice Soup

Prep Time: 15 minutes

Cook Time: 3 hours

Total Time: 3 hours 15 minutes

 Yield: 6

Ingredients

- cup dry (uncooked) wild rice
- lb boneless, skinless chicken breast
- ¼ cup olive oil, butter, ghee or vegan butter
- 5 cloves garlic, minced
- 1 cup chopped yellow onion
- 3/4 cup chopped celery
- 3/4 cup chopped carrots
- 1 teaspoon dried thyme
- 1 teaspoon dried rosemary
- teaspoons sea salt
- bay leaves
- 6 cups low sodium chicken broth
- cups water (or additional chicken broth)
- 1/2 cup gluten-free all purpose flour

- 1 cup unsweetened oat or almond milk
- sea salt and pepper to taste
- fresh thyme, for garnish (optional)

Instructions

1. Rinse the rice under running water. Place the uncooked rice, chicken breast, garlic, onions, celery, carrots, thyme, rosemary, salt, bay leaves, chicken broth and water into your slow cooker.

2. Cover and cook on the high setting for 3-4 hours or on the low setting for 7-8 hours. In the last 1/2 hour of cooking, remove the chicken from the slow cooker. Allow to cool slightly and then use two forks to shred the chicken into small pieces.

3. When the rice is done cooking, remove the bay leaves and add the shredded chicken back into the slow cooker. Melt the butter or oil in a saucepan. Add the flour and let the mixture cook for 1 minute. Whisk the mixture slowly while adding in the milk. Continue to whisk until all lumps have dissolved. Allow the mixture to thicken and become creamy.

4. Add the creamy mixture into the slow cooker. Stir to combine. Add additional water or milk to your preference if the consistency is too thick. Taste and season with salt and pepper if needed. Garnish with fresh thyme and serve.

25. Dairy-Free Spinach Quiche

Prep Time: 15 minutes

Cook Time: 52 minutes

Total Time: 1 hour 7 minutes

Yield: 8

Ingredients

(9-inch) pie crust (gluten-free, if needed)

- ½ teaspoon olive or avocado oil
- onion, chopped
- cloves of garlic, minced
- 1 cup chopped red, yellow or orange bell pepper
- teaspoons dried Italian seasoning
- 8–10 oz frozen chopped spinach, thawed and drained
- 1 teaspoon sea salt, to taste
- ¼ teaspoon freshly ground black pepper, to taste
- large eggs
- 1/3 cup egg whites (or 3 additional eggs)
- 2/3 cup unsweetened oat milk (or other non-dairy milk)

- Tablespoons nutritional yeast
- fresh chopped thyme, for garnish

Instructions

1. Preheat oven to 400°F.

2. All oil to a medium skillet over medium-high. Add onion, garlic, bell pepper and cook until onion is translucent, about 6-7 minutes. If you're using fresh spinach, after about 5 minutes add in your chopped spinach until cooked down. Sprinkle salt and pepper on veggies while they cook. Set aside to cool.

3. While the veggies cook, make sure the spinach is as dry as possible by squeezing out all of the water. I like wrapping the spinach in a couple paper towels while squeezing to help absorb some of the liquid.

4. In a small bowl, whisk together eggs, egg whites, oat milk, Italian seasoning and nutritional yeast. Scatter veggie mixture and chopped spinach on the bottom of prepared crust.

5. Pour egg mixture over top and push under any ingredients not covered by the egg mixture to prevent burning. Bake uncovered until set and golden brown around edges, about 45 minutes. Let quiche rest at room temperature for 10 minutes, then cut into slices, top with fresh thyme and serve.

6. Store leftovers in the fridge for up to 5 days. Reheat in the oven or toaster oven.

26. Spaghetti Squash Taco Bake

Prep Time: 10 minutes

 Cook Time: 35 minutes

Total Time: 45 minutes

Yield: 4

Ingredients

- spaghetti squash, roasted
- Tablespoon olive oil
- ½ yellow onion, chopped
- cloves garlic, minced
- 1 pound ground turkey
- Tablespoons taco seasoning
- 1 cup black beans, drained and rinsed
- ¼ cup salsa
- ¼ cup fresh chopped cilantro + more for garnish
- Tablespoons tomato paste
- 1 Tablespoon chopped jalapeño + more for garnish
- ½ teaspoon chili powder
- ¼ teaspoon pepper
- ¼ teaspoon sea salt

- 1 cup shredded Mexican cheese
- Toppings: green onions, avocado, plain Greek yogurt/sour cream, cilantro, jalapeño

Instructions

1. Roast spaghetti squash. (Instructions for how to cook spaghetti squash can be found here.)

2. While squash is roasting, heat oil in a large sauté pan over medium heat. Add onion and garlic and cook until fragrant, about 4-5 minutes. Add ground turkey and taco seasoning to the pan and cook, breaking meat apart with your spatula. Once turkey is cooked through and no longer pink, add black beans, salsa, cilantro, tomato paste, jalapeño, chili powder, pepper and sea salt to the pan. Stir until combined. Remove from heat and set aside.

3. One squash is roasted and cool enough to touch, remove spaghetti strands from the peel and add the squash to the pan with ground turkey mixture. Toss to combine then transfer to a 8×8 or 9×9 square baking dish. Sprinkle cheese on top.

4. Bake in the oven for 15-20 minutes at 375°F, or until spaghetti squash bake is warm throughout and cheese is melted.

5. Serve topped with fresh cilantro, jalapeño, green onions, chopped tomatoes, avocado and/or sour cream.

27. White Bean Chicken Chili

Prep Time: 15 minutes

Cook Time: 30 minutes

Total Time: 45 minutes

Yield: 6

Ingredients

- Tablespoon olive or avocado oil
- cloves garlic, minced
- yellow onion, diced
- ½–1 jalapeño, seeded and diced
- 1 teaspoon dried oregano
- 1 teaspoon ground cumin
- teaspoons chili powder
- 1 teaspoon sea salt
- ¼ teaspoon ground pepper
- (4 oz) cans mild diced green chiles
- 1 lb boneless skinless chicken breasts
- cups low-sodium chicken broth
- (15 oz) cans cannellini beans, drained and rinsed
- 1 1/2 cup frozen corn (no need to thaw)

- chopped cilantro, green onion, jalapeño and/or avocado, for garnish
- cornbread or tortilla chips, for serving

Instructions

1. Heat oil in a large pot over medium heat. Add garlic, onion and jalapeño and cook until soft and fragrant, about 5-6 minutes. Add oregano, cumin, chili powder and cook about 1 minute more. Add green chiles, chicken, and broth and season with salt and pepper.

2. Bring mixture to a boil, then reduce heat and simmer, covered for about 10 to 15 minutes, until chicken is tender and cooked through.

3. Use a fork or tongs to remove chicken from the soup, place on a plate and shred with two forks.

4. Place shredded chicken back in the pot and add beans and corn. Bring soup to a simmer and let cook another 10 minutes. Taste soup at this point and season with additional sea salt and pepper if needed.

5. Portion chili into bowls and garnish with chopped cilantro, green onion, extra jalapeño and/or avocado.
6. This chili is great served with tortilla chips or cornbread.

28. Mattar Tofu

Prep Time: 10 minutes

Cook Time: 20 minutes

Total Time: 30 minutes

Yield: 2

Ingredients

- (14 oz) package organic extra-firm tofu, cut into small cubes
- 1/2 Tablespoons coconut oil
- 1 inch piece of fresh ginger
- 1 clove fresh garlic, minced
- 1 medium yellow onion, chopped
- 1/4–1/2 teaspoon cayenne pepper
- 1/3 cup water
- 1/2 Tablespoon garam masala
- 1/2 Tablespoon ground coriander
- 1/4 teaspoon ground turmeric
- 1 teaspoon salt
- 1/8 teaspoon black pepper
- 1 (14 oz) can diced tomatoes with juice

- 1/2 cup vegetable broth
- 1 bag (2 cups) frozen baby peas, thawed slightly
- fresh chopped cilantro, for topping (optional)
- rice or cauliflower rice, for serving

Instructions

1. Place onion, ginger, garlic and cayenne pepper into the container of a blender or food processor along with 1/3 cup water and blend until the mixture turns into a smooth paste. Set aside.

2. Heat coconut oil in a large sauté pan. Once hot add tofu cubes in a single layer and stir-fry until golden. This shouldn't take very long. Once golden place tofu cubes onto a plate and set aside.

3. Carefully add the contents of the blender into the same sauté pan you used for the tofu. Just be very careful with this part as the paste may splatter. Cook, stirring constantly until the paste turns a light brown color (about 5-6 minutes).

4. Add the garam masala, coriander, turmeric, salt, pepper and tomatoes. Stir and cook for a few minutes

longer. Add in vegetable broth and peas, mix well and bring mixture to a boil.

5. Cover, lower heat and simmer gently for 10 minutes. Lift cover and add the tofu cubes. Simmer ten minutes or until tofu and peas are heated through. Top with a little cilantro and serve with brown, basmati, jasmine or cauliflower rice.

29. Soba Noodle Salad

Prep Time: 15 minutes

Cook Time: 15 minutes

Total Time: 30 minutes

Yield: 6

Ingredients

- medium red bell pepper, thinly sliced
- 2/3 cup red cabbage, roughly chopped
- small crowns (or 1 medium-large crown) of broccoli, broken into small florets
- (8 oz.) package of soba noodles
- 1 (16 oz.) package of frozen shelled edamame
- sesame seeds or Gomasio, to taste

Spicy Miso Sauce:

- 2 cloves garlic
- teaspoon grated fresh ginger
- juice of 2 limes
- Tablespoons unseasoned rice vinegar
- 1/2 Tablespoons maple syrup

- 1 Tablespoon white miso

- 1 Tablespoon peanut butter

- 1 Tablespoon sesame oil

- 1/2–1 Tablespoon sambal oelek (or other crushed chili paste)

- teaspoons bragg's liquid aminos (or low sodium soy sauce)

- 1/4 cup water, to thin

Instructions

1. Prep red bell pepper, red cabbage and broccoli by washing and chopping it.

2. Combine all ingredients for the sauce in a blender, blend and then set aside.

3. Begin cooking soba noodles according to package directions in a large pot. When you have about 5 minutes left, add the shelled edamame to the pot of cooking noodles. Place noodles and edamame in a colander and rinse with warm water, drain and place back into the pot. Add red cabbage on top of noodles.

4. While noodles (and edamame) are cooking, heat a large nonstick skillet over medium-high heat. Add 1/2 tablespoon coconut oil to pan; swirl to coat. Add red pepper and broccoli to pan; sauté 6-10 minutes or until tender.

5. Once the veggies are cooked to your liking, add them to the pot with the noodles, edamame and cabbage. Pour sauce over the mixture. Mix well to make sure the sauce gets distributed evenly. It's a little difficult to stir the noodles, but it's totally possible — just keep mixing.

6. Serve in plates or bowls, making sure to get a good mixture of noodles, edamame and veggies on each. Top with a sprinkle of sesame seeds or Gomasio. Enjoy!

30. Cheesy Cauliflower Nachos

Prep Time: 15 minutes

Cook Time: 27 minutes

Total Time: 42 minutes

Yield: 6

Ingredients

- Tablespoon olive or avocado oil
- 1/2 teaspoon garlic powder
- 1/2 teaspoon onion powder
- 1/2 teaspoon ground cumin
- 1/2 teaspoon paprika
- 1/4 teaspoon chili powder
- 1/2 teaspoon sea salt
- 5 cups cauliflower florets, cut into ½-inch slices
- 1/3 cup refried beans
- 3/4 cup shredded Mexican cheddar cheese
- jalapeno, sliced
- 1/2 cup chopped grape/cherry tomatoes
- 1/4 cup diced red onion
- 1/4 cup chopped fresh cilantro

- 1 avocado, sliced or chopped (optional)

Instructions

1. Preheat oven to 425°F. Spray a large baking sheet with olive oil or avocado oil cooking spray.

2. Slice cauliflower into 1/2-inch slices.

3. In a large bowl, combine oil with garlic powder, onion powder, cumin, paprika, chili powder and sea salt. Add sliced cauliflower and gently toss to coat. Place seasoned cauliflower on baking sheet, spacing out the pieces so that they roast instead of steam. Bake 20 minutes, until cauliflower is tender and starting to brown.

4. Remove the pan from the oven; push cauliflower together in the center of the pan. Top cauliflower with refried beans, sprinkle with cheese and add jalapeño slices on top. Return to the oven and bake until the beans are heated through and the cheese has melted, about 6-7 minutes.

www.ingramcontent.com/pod-product-compliance
Lightning Source LLC
Chambersburg PA
CBHW061723250726

48657CB00002B/741